Easy Weight Loss!

52 Easy Ways to Lose
Weight and Keep it Off!

By

Kimberly Peters

Also Available from 26Ways.com:

26 Ways to Get More Fun from
RC Aircraft

26 Ways to Save Money on
Your Utility Bills

26 Ways to Manage Your
Type 2 Diabetes & Control
Your Blood sugar

26 Ways to Become
A Better Manager

26 Ways to Grow Your
On-Line Business

26 Ways to Be the Best Wife Ever!

How to Retire Happy & Financially Secure

For all other Publications,
and for more information on our
books and manuals, please visit our
website at:

http://www.26ways.com

Contents

Disclaimer

The information provided in this book is intended for information purposes only and is not intended, nor should it be used, as a program or guide to treat or address any specific situation or individual. Everyone is different and some or all parts of this book may not be applicable to any individual. The writers, publishers and distributors of this title assume no responsibility for the use or application of any or all parts of this publication. The reader assumes all responsibility for determining the suitability of any part of this book as it pertains to their own situation. A doctor's approval is suggested before starting any weight loss or exercise program. We are not doctors and therefore offer no specific medical advice or opinions.

Introduction

When it comes to losing weight, this is something many people struggle with for most of their lives. Whether it is a few extra pounds that needs to come off to fit into that wedding dress or a hundred pounds that you need to lose to address or prevent medical problems, weight loss is rarely easy for most of us.

Though much has changed over the last hundred years, some things have pretty much stayed the same. We have technology now that we never would have dreamed on 50 years ago and our standard of living and quality of life has never been better either. But despite those changes losing weight still requires pretty much the same effort for most of us.

The great thing concerning weight loss is that we understand much more about it these days especially for people who gain weight for medical reasons or conditions. For those people our physicians and the medical community have more resources than ever before.

If you are one of these individuals, you should really check with your doctor about what options are available to you.

But for the rest of us, the weight loss process remains pretty much unchanged. Granted we have weight loss pills and supplements and there are more exercise gizmos, gyms and health clubs and more information available to us. But despite all of those things, if you want to lose weight you have to use more calories during the day than you take in. That is the simple truth.

One bad part of society today is that there are people and companies out there who look for people's weak spots or problems and then create products and services that are over advertised and hyped up just to get people to part with their hard earned money.

We have all seen those "lose weight in your sleep" or "lose 20 pounds in 20 days without diet and exercise" but with many of those products or programs the only thing that gets lighter is your wallet. But there are some good resources out there for you and you are either holding one or reading one right now.

Throughout this book we are going to concentrate on just one thing. That is how you can lose weight and keep it off while reducing the sacrifice and effort required to accomplish that goal. We believe that this can be accomplished if you just do a few important things and change an attitude or two along the way.

This book has two parts. The first part is some general information regarding weight loss that is important for everyone to know. This forms the basis for the second part of the book which deals with over 52 things anyone can do to help them lose the weight and then keep it off.

Many people struggle today not with just losing the weight but also keeping that weight off after they lose it. Commonly called "yo-yo dieting" this refers to people losing weight, gaining it back then losing it again and then gaining it back over and over and over again. Not only is this frustrating but it can be unhealthy as well. That is why the first part of this book is so important so please do not by pass this part because you think you already know it. Sometimes understanding something in a different light can bring everything into focus for you.

The second part of the book is the 52 ways to lose weight and the focal point of the book. These are the things you can do in order to make weight loss easier and possibly faster. This is important because we all know that if we make something easier, or if we can get positive results faster, we will keep doing those things for longer periods of time. This doesn't mean we are lazy, it just means we usually cannot sustain a large effort for long periods of time.

As you go through these 52 tips and techniques, you are going to read information that you have read before. This is not s mistake but done on purpose for three reasons.

First, some concepts have certain things in common with other concepts so the descriptions might contain information you previously read. Second, some people don't read a book from page one until the end. They skip around. When people skip around, they read things out of order and if a piece of information is left out because it was discussed previously, then that person might not fully understand what they are reading. With this book you can start at the beginning or with tip 38 and you will be fine.

Finally, some information is just so important or critical that you need to hear it multiple times so that you pay attention to it and understand its importance. Plus, repetition allows you to retain information longer and the really important information needs to be remembered longer than some of the other things you might read.

Just because there are 52 tips doesn't mean you have to do all 52 in order to be successful and lose weight. You might only need one or two to make a difference. Or you might need 15 or 20! Only you can determine what you need in order to achieve your goal. We have given you the toolbox, you just need to pick out the tools you need for this project.

Some of these tools might not apply to you or you are already using them and that's perfectly fine. Rarely do we have someone who needs all 52 so just start by picking the one or two that you think will give you the biggest benefits and get started. As we say in the book, if you don't change anything, nothing changes!

Now for the first thing you will read that is repeated several times throughout this book. Please take this to heart because it is extremely important.

Before you start any weight loss program PLEASE see your doctor and go over your plan with him or her. They can advise you on what is appropriate and give you any limits or restrictions on your weight loss program. This is important because everyone is different and what works for one person might be really bad for someone else. Please check with your doctor and work out a healthy program with them.

Now, let's start making some changes!

Why Do You Want
to Lose Weight?

I am assuming that because you opened this book that you want to lose weight. It really doesn't matter what the reason for this weight loss might be as long as it is YOU that wants to lose it. Because if you are doing something because someone else wants you to that can be very difficult.

You need to understand the reasons for wanting to lose weight. Do you want to look better, feel better or make something in your life better? Do you want to be able to do certain things that you cannot do now because of excess weight or lack of energy? Whatever those reasons might be, they have to be your reasons.

The only exception to this rule might be when your doctor tells you that you need to lose weight for a medical reason. Maybe you are at risk for a disease such as diabetes or maybe you already have diabetes. Maybe your blood pressure is too high because of the extra pounds. If that is the reason for your desire to lose weight then those reasons need to become YOUR reasons. You need to understand them, believe them and make them your reasons.

Once you know the reasons behind wanting to lose weight, you need to visualize how life will be once you lose the weight. Will you feel better? Will you look better? Will you have more energy or be able to do more or different things? Visualize how your life will be better once you lose that weight.

This will provide you with constant motivation throughout the weight loss process. You will use this motivation to help you stay with the program and remain committed to your weight loss goals. Weight loss is not a one day or one month process. It goes on for a while and you need to remain engaged and motivated throughout the entire process.

Motivation is much easier when it is YOU that wants to achieve that goal. You might want to make a spouse or loved one happy by losing weight but that is not the same as wanting it for your own reasons and for yourself.

So take a few moments to really understand why you want to lose weight and how life will be after you lose that weight. Be specific and as detailed as you can be. Picture life like it will be in vivid detail. Create bright and detailed pictures in your mind that are so real you can almost touch and feel them.

Then go out and turn those pictures into reality.

Your Weight Loss Goals

We all have goals in life whether they pertain to weight loss, career, relationships or any other part of our lives. Goals help us turn desires into our reality. They provide a target to shoot for or something to accomplish. Goals add dimension to what we feel and help us make them real. They also help us understand what needs to be done.

Specific goals are much better and far more motivating. They also provide better results. Make your goals as specific as possible. Change "I want to lose weight" into "I want to lose 15 pounds." This will not only tell you that you want to lose weight but exactly how much. You will know what is involved and what needs to be done. You will have a deeper understanding of the task at hand and what needs to be done to achieve it.

Also, give your goals a time frame. Even "I want to lose 15 pounds" is not a good goal if you don't give yourself a time frame in which to achieve it.

If you took 50 years to lose those 15 pounds would that be achieving your goal? Technically, it would be because you provided no time frame. But a goals such as "I want to lose 15 pound this year" or "I want to lose 15 pounds in 6 months" would give you both a target figure as well as a time frame in which you want to achieve it.

Time frames help you determine what needs to be done more accurately. After all it would require different techniques to lose that 15 pounds in 6 months than it would to lose that same weight in 50 years! The more accurately and specifically your goal is, the more likely you will be to achieve it.

Perhaps the most important aspect of a goal is that it be realistic and achievable. If you set a goal so high that you cannot possibly achieve it then all you are doing is setting yourself up for confusion and frustration. If you set a goal to lose 30 pounds in one month, you are setting yourself up to fail. You just cannot accomplish that kind of goal in a healthy manner unless it involves surgery or other similar intervention.

Your goals should be realistic and they should be set in such a manner that they can be achieved in a healthy and responsible manner. You should not be starving yourself or working out 20 hours a day to achieve an overly ambitious goal.

Set your goals with the help of your doctor or trainer and make them achievable. Achievable goals will keep you engaged and motivated far longer than ridiculous goals.

You should always understand that goals are never etched in stone unless there are specific reasons that they need to be. In other words, you can set a goal and adjust it over time. For example, you can set a goal of losing 15 pounds in 6 months and then adjust it to 20 pounds if you hit the 15 pounds in 4 months. Or, if things were harder than you originally thought, you might make that 10 pounds in 6 months or 15 pounds in one year.

Goals are designed to help you focus on your goals and achieve them. Goals are for you and yourself only. You do not have to get others involved unless you want to. You should be setting your goals so that you can achieve the desired result. The only exception might be if your weight loss is tied to a medical condition which requires a specific weight loss goal within a specific time frame. Even then you would work with your doctor and adjust your goals over time.

Last, but certainly not least, don't set your goals based on what others have achieved or what others have set as their goals. Everyone is different and everyone needs to have their own goals and their own objectives. Just because Bob in accounting lost 15 pounds in 2 months doesn't mean that is achievable or desirable for you. You are not Bob, you are you!

So let's arrive at some specific goals, assign those goals a time frame and then figure out an action plan designed to achieve those goals. That is the first step but it is an important step. Having a set goal and a plan to achieve it almost always achieves better results in far less time.

Your Environment

Before we get started on trying to figure out the best way for us to lose the weight we need to lose, let's talk about how our environment not only influences how much we eat, what we eat and why we eat.

There are various parts of our environment that will have a direct impact on how successful we are in losing weight. Here are just a few of the most common environmental factors as they apply to weight gain or loss:

Available Foods

One of the most common problems people trying to lose weight encounter are the foods that they find around them. While we can control what we have at home, when we are at work or outside we often are tempted or distracted by other foods. People bring snacks into work or we go out to eat and the portions are huge and the calories sky high.

But the foods we have in our own home often represent that greatest challenge. If we purchase foods that are high in calories, or if they are very easy to get, we will be more likely to eat them. So it makes sense to try and keep temptation away by not keeping those items in our home.

People

If we live by ourselves then keeping high calorie foods away is as easy as not buying them in the first place. But when we live with others whether they might be friends, family or kinds, we cannot and should not expect others to stop eating what they enjoy because we do not wish to be tempted.

Plus other people want to eat what they want and often they will do that in our presence. Friends and co-workers are prime example of this. They will eat high calorie or comfort food around you and that can be tempting as well.

Peer pressure can be very strong as well. We always want to fit in and be like everyone else so when everyone is going out to the burger joint for lunch we do not want to stay back and eat our salad. Or even when we do join everyone else we don't want to be the only one not having a burger but eating a salad instead. This can lead to ridicule or being made fun of.

Then there are those people who seem to make it a life mission to get you to stop trying to lose weight. Maybe they are overweight themselves and haven't been able to lose the weight. Maybe they are threatened by you in some way and want to see you fail. Or, they could just have their own reasons or agenda when it comes to you and your weight loss. After all, we all know people who are just mean for what seems like no reason at all.

Schedule

People seem to be a lot busier these days and busy schedules often mean grabbing meals and food on the run. That usually means fast food or grabbing a sandwich or other high calorie foods instead of healthy choices.

While I understand why this happens, there are many alternatives to fast food if we really want to stop buying it. But they require time to prepare and a little bit of thought and planning so that you have it handy when you need it.

If your job has you in an office you can bring in meals from home for lunch instead of going out. But if you are on the road and have to eat several meals out, then that can present a challenge for almost everyone. If that is your situation, you will need to take care of some extra planning to accommodate your meals during the week.

Local Area

When I was growing up, we had a diner, an ice cream store and a donut shop nearby. But today, in my town there are 8 different fast food places, 4 theme restaurants, several convenience stores, 3 different ice cream places and untold pizza places. Most of these are within walking distance.

The point I am trying to make is that comfort food and fast food as so much easier to get today. That is why our children and others are getting more and more obese. There is little effort required to get this type of food. So it becomes a larger part of our diet than it should be. As we mentioned before with schedules, this type of food is so convenient we often sacrifice nutrition for speed and convenience.

Creating the Best Environment

Several of the tips we are going to give you concern creating a better weight loss environment so we will not get into specifics at this point. But I want you to think of your environment now and break it down into two parts.

The first part are the things that support your weight loss and help you in your efforts to lose weight. These are the parts of your environment that will help bring you closer to your goals.

These would include supportive people, healthy choices for food and meals and other things that help make it easier to develop a healthier lifestyle.

These are the things that we need to make a larger part of our lives. These are the parts of our environment that help keep us motivated and make it easier to do the right things. Sometimes intentions are just not good enough. We need convenience and making things easier so that we keep on doing the right things. So take the positive parts of our environment and make them a larger part of our life.

The second part are the things that make our efforts more difficult or even impossible. These might be the people who are always trying to get us to eat "bad foods" or tempting us with things that aren't good for us. Every environment has things that help take us away from our goals and what we really want. These are the things that we need to stay away from in our life.

That might mean staying away from certain people, taking a different route home from work so you are not driving by the fast food or ice cream stores. It might mean dealing with destructive or negative people so that they are more aware of what they are doing and why it should stop.

Your environment is a crucial part of your overall success or failure. Desire and intentions play a role in getting you started but they are only temporary motivators.

Will power is a myth as well. If we don't eliminate or at least reduce temptation and surround us with positive role models and surroundings, we will eventually fail.

I do not say this to be negative or to discourage anyone. To the contrary, I am telling you this now so you can start to identify negative influences and areas of your environment NOW and take action so that once you get started there will be far fewer things in your way.

Just do not discount the importance of creating the most positive environment so that it will help push you towards your goals and not away from them.

What Works for You?

Whenever we want to accomplish something or look for better ways to do things, we often look to see what has worked for other people. After all, it makes sense that if something worked for one person it could work for us as well. But when it comes to losing weight, an individualized approach is usually best.

You own overall health, age and other factors might make it impossible for you to do what worked for other people. There are many factors that go into what is the best way to lose weight. But regardless of your personal situation, there are rules and guidelines everyone trying to lose weight needs to follow.

Here are a few of those common rules:

See Your Doctor

You are going to read this several times throughout this book because this is one of the most important parts of any weight loss program. Any time we change what goes in our bodies or we change what we expect our bodies to do, we should consult our doctor for their approval.

This is especially true if we are getting on in years or if we have any diseases or medical conditions that might be effected by dieting or exercise. In these cases you doctor will advise you on what you can and cannot do as well as a schedule for when to safely increase your exercise levels.

At minimum you should get a yearly physical and discuss your weight goals before you start to make sure they are reasonable and healthy goals for you personally. This is important because what's healthy for you and what's healthy for Cousin Ed or Uncle Bob could be totally different.

If you are planning on taking any weight loss drugs or supplements, get your doctor's approval before taking them. This is even more important if you are on any other medications because there could be interaction between the medications and supplements. It is better to be safe than sorry.

Take the Healthy Approach

Sometimes we might be tempted to get results fast instead of taking the healthy road. Do not do that. Make sure your plan is medically sound and that your diet gives your body everything it needs to function properly and maintain a high level of health.

This means eating right and not starving yourself. It means getting the right amount of exercise and the appropriate type of exercise for you age and physical condition. It means not trying to take short-cuts with pills or supplements that are not proven or accepted by your doctor.

It also means losing weight at a healthy and responsible pace. Slow and steady weight loss is almost always preferable and more desirable by your doctor. It is not important how long it takes to get to your goal as long as you get to it eventually. It might take a month or it might take two years if you have a lot of weight to lose. Don't rush things. Keep it healthy.

Know Your Limitations

The days of going all out and not worrying about health and safety are probably long gone for you. Even if you are only in your 20's you are not the same as you were when you were 10. You need to understand that and be honest with yourself when it comes to what you can, cannot and should not do when it comes to weight loss.

For example, don't try to lift 150 pounds when you can only safely lift 50 pounds. Don't try to run a marathon if you never ran more than a tenth of a mile before. Don't try and convince yourself that you can do something you know you can't. This is one time when mind over matter just doesn't apply!

Create a Plan You Can Stick With

The thing about crash diets and quick weight loss plans is that they require a LOT of effort and sacrifice. You might be capable of doing this for a short time while the novelty of the process is still new and when you see the greatest results. But when weight loss slows down a bit, you are going to lose motivation.

It is much better to create an easier plan that will allow you to lose weight the best way for you. That means doing the exercises you enjoy, playing the sports you love and eating the foods you like instead of whatever those "canned diets" might tell you. If you enjoy playing basketball then get your cardio on the basketball court. If you like to eat chicken then bake yourself some chicken. The more we enjoy what we are doing the far more likely it is that you will continue the effort. You will hear more about this throughout this book.

Start Slow & Work Gradually

Losing weight requires a change in diet or exercise. But we want to be smart and take the healthy approach which means starting slowly and gradually building top our maximum effort. Cutting down gradually on what we eat and gradually increasing our exercise levels allows our bodies a chance to adapt to your new lifestyle.

This is not only a healthier way of approaching weight loss but it is a safer way as well. Gradually starting to exercise gives our bodies a chance to get used to the new physical activity without straining or damaging our muscles. A little muscle soreness is OK and an indication that you are using your muscles more than you are used to. But a visit to the emergency room or not being able to walk the next morning signal you did too much, too soon!

Remember your goal is to find something you can do for extended periods of time. Gradually starting exercise will spare you the pain and torture and provide you with something you can stick with even after you have lost the weight you wanted to lose!

Do What Works for You NOT Anyone Else!

Always remember that you are you and that you are different than anyone else. That means certain things will work better than others will for you. It might be different for someone else but we are not losing weight for someone else. We are losing weight for US!

There are well over 50 tips in this book. Some will work well for you while others you might not even want to consider. This doesn't mean you have failed or are not worthy of making the effort. What it does mean is that you were smart enough to realize that certain things just are not a good mix for you. Stick with what you feel will work best for you and not what worked for someone else!

So now we are ready to get started. Take it slow and be smart throughout the process. Expect more of yourself but not too much. This is always going to be a work in progress and changes will be made to help move things along.

The best part is that you pushed yourself to get to this point. You understand that there is something you want to accomplish and you are making the effort to accomplish it on your terms. You should be commended for that because that is going further than a lot of people get.

Medical Intervention

Though we are not medical experts, and though this is not part of the focus of this book, since there often is a medical component to weight gain and loss we figured we should address the need for medical intervention when it becomes necessary. Again, we are not doctors nor do we have any medical training. You should refer to your doctor for all medical related issues and questions pertaining to weight loss.

Sometimes the need for extreme weight loss for health reasons might require medical intervention. This might mean surgical procedures or the use of prescriptions medications designed to assist in the weight loss process. This is usually done when the weight loss is too great for someone to handle on their own or whenever there is medical reasons for a more controlled or rapid weight loss.

In other situations, weight gain can be caused by a medical condition which makes losing weight difficult if not impossible.

In order to confirm that a medical condition is the reason for your weight gain or inability to lose weight, you will need to have a thorough evaluation by a medical professional. Your family doctor can do this or can send you to a qualified doctor specializing in that field or those diseases. This is NOT something that can be decided by the patient alone. They MUST get examined and evaluated first.

All weight loss drugs and / or procedures should be approved and recommended by your doctor. You should not be deciding on your own what the best course of action is. This is especially true if you are currently taking other medications as there can be interaction between medications that could cause serious problems.

Your doctor will recommend a physician who specializes in weight loss to evaluate you and your present condition and suggest the possible alternatives for you. Whether or not your options include surgery or other procedures will be up to your doctor. Listen to what they tell you and discuss things to decide which the right option for you is.

You should be aware that medical intervention and surgery should only be reserved for those people who medically require it and not as a substitute for normal dieting and exercise. There are risks associated with any surgery or taking any medication so these decisions are best left up to trained medical professionals.

If you feel that your weight loss requires medical intervention, then schedule an appointment with your doctor to confirm medical intervention is indicated and to discuss your options.

Here are the 52 Ways to Lose the Weight You Want to Lose

1.   Drink More Water

Most of us don't drink enough water and that can be unhealthy all by itself. Still others refuse to drink more water because they think it makes them weigh more. But the fact is, if you drink more water you will lose more weight!

Think about this for a moment. When you drink more water, you make the body process more water. That takes energy which means your body is burning off more calories processing that extra water.

Another positive is that your body needs water to function properly and to be able to flush out toxins and other substances from the body. When you don't drink enough water you can cause all kinds of problems from kidney stones, urinary tract infections and other not so nice health problems.

From a weight loss perspective water helps you feel full after you drink it. If your stomach feels empty that sends a signal to your brain that you are hungry. Sometimes drinking a glass of water will make you feel fuller and reduce that craving to eat.

2. Change to Diet Soda to Water

Most of us today drink entirely too much soda. Soda is chocked full of sugar and can really help us pack on the pounds. Just one super-sized soda can have over 500 calories in it! That is over ¼ of the total calories we should be consuming in an entire day! If you really have to drink a soda, try to make it a small one and then even then only one or two times a week.

Even diet soda will help us pack on the pounds because of the artificial sweeteners and their effect on our bodies. Sometimes we even think that because the soda has no calories we can drink even more of it. The fact is there are no benefits to drinking soda and there is no nutritional value in it either.

We are much better off switching from diet soda to just plain old water. Water has zero calories, no artificial ingredients and no chemicals that can harm our bodies. Plus, as we have already stated water is a natural way to cleanse the body and remove impurities and waste products making us feel better and healthier in the process.

3. Drink Water Before a Meal

Drinking water before every meal can help us fill up a little bit of our stomach so that we get that full feeling a bit faster. Not only that but water helps us digest our foods better and allows digestion to become easier and more efficient.

But if drinking a full glass of water allows us to eat a few bites less of food during the course of a meal, that can add up to the loss of several pounds of the course of a month or so. While water itself will not cause weight loss, eating less because we feel full most certainly will.

4.   Limit Alcoholic Beverages

Another area where we can really pack on the pound is in our consumption of alcoholic beverages. Alcoholic beverages can contain a load of calories and have limited health benefits as well.

If you are out at a restaurant or bar substitute club soda or seltzer for alcohol. Not only will you save a lot of calories it is always safe to drive under the influence of seltzer. Unless that is, you drank so much seltzer that you have to speed home to get to the bathroom!

5. Lite Beverages are NOT Calorie Free Beverages!

Sometimes when we drink a Lite Beer or reduced calorie drink we convince ourselves that we are drinking responsibly as far as calories are concerned so it is all right to drink twice as much. The fact is, lite beverages do have calories and sometimes the difference between the lite version and the regular version is not all that much.

While it is important to drink any kind of beverage, even lite beverages, responsibly, we should always remember that lite beer still has alcohol in it and alcohol still contains calories and can still influence our driving and cognitive functions.

So even if weight loss is not a chief concern of yours it still makes sense to switch to seltzer or water whenever you are drinking out. You will save calories, make better overall decisions and be healthier in the process. I know I sound like your mother but I really do speak the truth!

6. Exercise in Moderation

We all equate weight loss with exercise and for good reason. Most of us will not be able to lose the weight by just diet alone.

We are going to need a combination of diet and exercise to get the job done.

But a lot of us make one very bad mistake. We think that in order to be beneficial, we have to work out like mad men, run a marathon, lift 500 pound weights and all that other crap. The reality is though that we don't have to do any of those thing in order to lose weight. We just have to exercise responsibly.

That means working up a sweat but not to the point where we ache and stain and do ourselves harm in the process. We need to start off slow and give our bodies a chance to get used to the exercise and then gradually increase the duration and/or intensity.

But even if our bodies can take it, our minds might not. We might hate exercising so much that we just stop doing it. The key is to exercise regularly at a pace and level that is enjoyable so we continue to exercise in the future. That means going twice a week or so for months not 5 times week for two weeks!

It means exercising to the point where we burn off calories but can still get out of bed the next day without feeling like a 90 year old! Like everything else in life, we need to achieve a balance between what works and what we can keep up with. Once we manage that, we are good to go!

7.   Get Some Cardio

Exercise is great but we also need some cardio exercise in order to get the weight loss process going. Again, like we said in the last item, we do not need to run a marathon or run at 10 miles an hour to see results. Instead we should strive for a certain amount of exercise every week.

The established rule of thumb is to exercise for at least 30 minutes straight 4 or 5 times a week. You need at least 30 minutes to enter the fat burning cycle and you need the frequency to keep the body burning fat. If you can do more than the 30 minutes that's great but try and exercise at least every other day and get that heart rate up!

Check with your doctor as far as how much exercise you can tolerate and what your maximum pulse rate should be. That will depend on your age and overall health condition. If you suffer from any diseases or physical ailments that will affect your maximum heart rate.

Try and hit a level where you are pushing yourself a bit but can still talk normally at the same time. If things are a bit much then slow down or reduce the intensity. Remember we need length as well as time so we need to balance both out.

Try running on a treadmill or around the neighborhood. Running is a good exercise as long as your body is up to it. If running is too strenuous, walking might be a better choice. Which is good because that is the next item on our list!

8.   Walk More

Walking is one of the easiest things that just about anyone can do at least to some extent. We can build it into our daily schedule in so many ways that we can burn extra calories without even realizing it.

Walking is not going to make you lose 20 pounds in a month but it also is not going to injure you either as long as you are careful. The key is to use moderation when it comes to starting anything new.

For example, if you are not used to walking a lot do not try and walk 10 miles the first time out. Go for a walk around the block or around a small part of the neighborhood. Allow you joints and body to get used to walking and then increase it slowly from there.

Even if you just burn an extra 50 calories a day, at the end of the year you will have burned over 18,000 calories which means if you changed nothing else whatsoever you would lose 5 pounds after one year just by walking and burning an additional 50 calories a day!

Do you think you could do that? I think you can! In fact, the next few tips are going to concentrate on easy ways that we can incorporate a little bit more walking into our lifestyle without causing stress or sweating too much!

9.   Park Further Away

The next time you go to the store or wherever you are going, park further away. Unless it is raining or snowing or bitter cold, park on the outer parts of the parking lot and walk those extra steps to and from the car. Leave those parking spots in the front of the store to people who might really need them.

This is a short-term exercise that will not help you as far as cardio is concerned but it will help you burn some extra calories and remember that is always our objective. To burn more calories without necessarily realizing it! So next time, park a bit further away from the store.

10. Walk around the Store While Shopping

Here is one that can really add up whenever you go shopping. When I go food shopping, or whenever I have to shop for more than one item, I get my first item, then I walk the perimeter of the store and then go for my second item.

I keep on doing this until all the items are in my cart. Then I take one last perimeter walk and head for the checkout.

This can really add up. It is not unusual for me to add about 2,000 steps to my daily total just by doing this simple technique. Sometimes people working at the store might ask you if you need help finding something because they see you walking so much but that is something I am willing to put up with.

11.   Walk While on the Phone

We all spend time talking on the phone and this can be better put to use by adding a little walking into our schedule at the same time. If we use a cordless phone and walk around the house while we are talking we can burn off more than a few calories while we are on the phone!

I often have conference calls at work and these can take up one or two hours or more. So using a cordless phone, I walk around the house or around my office and just keep moving. You would be surprised how much movement and how many calories you can add just by doing this.

The best part is that you don't even realize that you are moving. You are concentrating so much on the conversation that you forget you are moving and burning calories. Since this makes it easy, this is one of the best and easiest ways to add a little bit of movement and exercise into your daily schedule.

To make this even easier, see if your phone has a jack for a headset. If it does, then purchase an inexpensive headset to wear while you are moving around. This will make it easier to move your arms and your arm will not get tired from holding the phone to your ear. You could use a speakerphone but sometimes this is not the best way to hold a conversation with all the noises around you making it hard for the other person to hear.

If your phone does not have a headset or handset jack, look for a model that does when it comes time to replace your phone.

12.   Walking Instead of Driving

It is surprising when you realize just how many of the places we go or the things that we do are so close to home. Now if you live in a rural environment this might not apply to you but I find it very easy to accomplish some of my errands by walking instead of driving.

For example, well within walking distance of my home there is the library, drug store, card store, bagel store and a supermarket. So if I need to go to any of those places, and I don't have to pick up a lot of things, then I simply walk instead of driving.

The result is that although I take a little bit more time to accomplish things, I burn calories, get some cardio and save on gas as well.

Plus, I don't have to worry about getting a parking spot and I get a little bit of time outdoors which is good for you as well.

There are also a couple of fast food places that I enjoy as well so I can walk to one of them and even though the food isn't the healthiest or low calorie, I still burn off a few extra calories walking to and back from them. This is sort of a compromise where I get the food I crave while minimizing the negatives in getting it!

13.   Do Strength Training to Build Muscle

Let's get one thing straight. I do not like strength training. I wouldn't go so far as saying I hate it but I dislike it. But I am starting to change my opinion of it because I have noticed some very real benefits from doing it.

First, strength training builds muscle while burning off calories that reduce the fat in our bodies. So you are adding good muscle while removing bad fat. That's a win-win for us!

Second, muscle by itself burns more calories than fat does so the more muscle we have in our bodies the more calories we will burn for doing the same things every day. So creating muscle will help us burn more calories just maintaining that muscle!

You need to be careful when it comes to strength training, however.

I strongly urge you to consult with your doctor AND a personal trainer so that you can start healthy and not risk injury. Too many people are hurt trying to lift more than they are capable of. Stay within your capabilities and move up in weight only when you are able.

14.   Always Keep Moving

Movement requires energy and energy requires the burning of calories. Just moving constantly no matter what you are doing will help you burn more calories. You can watch television if you want but move while you do it. Move around, stretch out your muscles, stretch your back out, lift a small dumbbell or do anything that requires movement of any kind. Nervous or fidgety people are burning more calories than the rest of us.

Try and see what movements you can make while you go through your day. Every little thing helps and by the end of the day you can wind up with a lot extra bonus calories burned!

15.   Try Alternatives to Frying

Even healthy foods can become unhealthy if they are cooked certain ways. Frying our foods makes them have more calories and higher fat content. This can add up to 1,000's of extra calories without eating extra food!

Try baking or grilling foods to cut down on the fat and extra calories. Some foods might be good cooked with hot air or a convection oven instead of frying. If you have to fry any food try and cut down on the portion size to reduce the amount of calories you are taking in. Frying might taste better but it will cause you to either gain weight or reduce the amount you will lose.

16.   Don't Skip Meals

One of the common things people try to do to lose weight is to skip a meal during the day and eat two meals instead of three. While this might appear to make sense on the surface, they fact is that skipping meals usually ends in gaining weight not losing it. That happens for two main reasons.

First, when you skip a meal you are usually a lot hungrier when it comes time for your next meal so you tend to eat more. Usually you will eat more calories in the two meals than you would have eaten in the three normal meals.

Not only that but when you are hungry you also tend to snack more. A few crackers here, a candy bar there and a few sodas and you not only made up for that lost meal but have consumed a lot more "empty calories". These are calories with limited or no nutritional value.

Second, when you skip meals your body senses it is not getting the food it wants and it tends to place your body into a lower metabolism or fat storage mode to protect itself against what it perceives as a lack of food. So your body tends to store more of what you do eat as fat and it slows your metabolism even more.

A lower metabolism will cause you to burn fewer calories during all your activities so the result is you burn fewer calories every day. That means you will have to work harder to accomplish the same goals. So eat every normal scheduled meal to keep your metabolism revved up and your calorie burning at a high level.

17.   Eat More Slowly and Chew More

Digestion starts in the mouth so you should make it a habit to start the digestion process efficiently and properly. This means eating more slowly and chewing your food thoroughly. Eating slowly helps you lose weight because by keeping the food in your mouth longer you allow your brain to send messages that you are full more quickly. The result is that you will feel full faster and therefore eat less.

Eating faster also allows us to consume more food in less time and more food means more calories.

So we can overeat before we get the "I feel full" sensation and we will consume more calories.

Chewing more will also help our bodies digest food better and more efficiently. This will help the overall digestive process and that will help us in other ways as well. Chewing more will also help us burn more calories too.

18.   Clean out the Pantry and Fridge

If we have things within reach we are far more likely to eat them on a whim. That package of cookies is far more tempting than having to get in the car, drive to the store and buy those cookies. The more difficult we make it to eat the foods that are bad for us the more often we will eat them.

Go through the pantry and the refrigerator and freezer and toss out the high calorie foods we don't want to eat any more. Do this on a full stomach so you are not tempted to keep something because it looks so good. Even worse, if you do this when you are hungry you will be tempted to eat things that you might otherwise throw out!

Do your best to create a house full of healthy and low calorie food to replace those high calorie snacks and meals. If the stuff isn't there for you to eat you won't eat it. It is really as simple as that for many people.

19.   Share a Meal

If you like to go out to eat that can be difficult because in some restaurants the portions are so large there is no way you can eat all of what they give you and still have a prayer of losing weight. But that doesn't mean you have to avoid the enjoyment of going out to eat.

One particularly creative way of addressing this problem is to go out with a friend or two and share an entrée or appetizer. If two people share that 12 ounce burger, the result is that both people get a human sized burger which should be more than adequate for a meal.

Another option, if allowed, is to order off the children's menu. These are usually smaller sized versions of adult entrees. This might be a good way to go out and still limit calories.

20.   Hold the Chips & Bread When Out

One of the great things about going out to some restaurants is the bread or chips they serve you while you are waiting for your food to arrive. While a nice warm piece of bread can be tasty, it also contains a ton of calories and carbohydrates which can really add up.

Consider asking the waiter or waitress to not bring you the bread or chips. This will help you avoid the temptation of having the basket sitting there in front of you. Even just eating one small piece is not possible when the rest of the basket is just sitting in front of you the whole time.

Another why holding the bread and chips will help you reduce calorie intake is that when you have bread you usually [put butter on the bread. This is all fat and calories and can really add up those calories in a hurry! Those chips are usually fried and have sauce or salsa with tem as well. So hold the bread, chips and what goes on them for a low calorie meal out.

21. Measure out Servings in Advance

Sometimes we try to eat right and responsibly but we don't do something quite right or make the right judgments. One perfect example of this is staying within the correct portion size when we make a meal. We might "think" that we are eating one portion or serving when in fact we might be eating 1.5,2 or 3 servings instead! The more servings, the more calories and the less weight we lose.

Our eyes sometimes trick us into thinking that something is a certain size. That bowl of cereal might look like a cup when it really is a cup and a half. That doesn't sound like a lot but an extra 50 calories a day ends up being 1,500 calories a month and that's a half pound of weight right there!

Another reason is that sometimes we are just too busy, or it is inconvenient, to take out the measuring cups or spoons and measure out a real cup or tablespoon of something. We might be rushed at home or are eating at work where we don't have the spoons.

I SUGGEST MEASURING OUT PORTION SIZES IN ADVANCE WHENEVER POSSIBLE. Use a zip-lock bad or other storage container and, if the product will not go bad or spoil, measure out a week's worth of servings. If you eat cereal for breakfast, measure out a week's worth in bags and then every morning you just have to take out a bag and pour it into a bowl. If you are at work, you can leave the bags in your desk and use them whenever you want.

There is no real way we can believe our eyes when it comes to how much we are eating or pouring. We can come close after a little practice but every little bit more we eat adds up. Plus, if we put a little bit more in the bowl every day eventually that tends to look normal and then we risk adding even more to the bowl every day.

You want to lose weight and your attitude and intentions are great. Just protect your efforts and measuring out portion size so there is no doubt you are eating the amount you want to eat and not a bit more or less.

22. Get Your Daily Amount of Quality Sleep

The human body reacts to different things in unexpected ways. One of those reactions comes from not getting enough sleep. Lack of sleep effects your metabolism and that can lead directly to added pounds.

Though the "normal" amount of sleep is usually considered to be 8 hours, everyone is different and you might function perfectly on 6 hours or you might require 10 hours. Only you can tell how refreshed and ready you feel to start the day each morning. If you feel fine in the morning but crash at noontime, you might need a bit of extra sleep during the night to stop mid-day crashes.

Quality of sleep is important as well. A good and restful night's sleep allows your body to recover from the previous day and to rebuild muscles and heal itself so you are ready to take on a new day tomorrow. Just lying in bed wide awake or having a fitful or restless night's sleep is not the same thing.

Another reason that sleep is important is that sometimes our busy schedules require more awake time each day as we try to fit more and more into a single day. Sometimes because we want to and sometimes because we have to. But when our schedules get so busy and rushed, we usually resort to fast food or grabbing snacks on the go and these are usually the high calorie type of food we should avoid.

So get your sleep, eat right and listen to your body throughout the day.

23.   Weigh Yourself Regularly

OK, this is where some people might disagree but I personally think we should weigh ourselves regularly. By regularly I mean once a day. I think this is the right approach for two very important reasons.

First, seeing the weight drop off motivates us to continue what we are doing. If we see ourselves dropping weight every day, or most days, we might be better able to resist getting that ice cream sundae and instead have some yogurt. When it comes to losing weight constant motivation is HUGE!

Second, should we have a bad day and gain a bit of weight, we find out about it NOW rather than continuing to do the same thing for a week and then see a LOT more weight on the scale. This way we can monitor things on a daily basis and catch problems or weight gains earlier when they are smaller.

Now this does not mean you need to weigh yourself 10 times a day. I would think once a day should be adequate. There are too many different things we do during the day that can make us gain or lose weight temporarily to make weighing ourselves several times a day pretty much useless.

But when you weight yourself every day, try and weigh yourself around the same time every day. Our weight can fluctuate a few pounds from morning to night so if you are going to compare weights, compare them at the same time as well. We usually weight less in the morning that we do at night.

24. Don't Eat for Comfort

As I am wringing this tip I am shaking my head because this is something I have done, and will probably continue to do to some extent, all my life. I tend to eat as a form of winding down or when things get a little bit tense or negative. You know what I'm talking about. You have a bad day at work so you stop for a few drinks and a plate of wings, or you hit a restaurant for a really good burger to help take your mind off of things.

This is something we have been programmed to do almost since birth for some of us. When we were younger and we were sad or upset, Mom gave us a piece of cake or a cookie or piece of candy. Something bad happen, take the kids for ice cream or a fast food splurge. It is what advertising and people have programmed each other to do for years.

But make no mistake about it. Food's primary function and purpose in life is for nourishment and to sustain life.

Food is eaten to provide nourishment so our bodies can continue to function at the right levels. So it is important to keep that in mind when you choose to eat and what to eat.

If you are angry or upset, try and come up with a different response. If you are angry, try taking a walk or going to the gym to burn off that anger. Do not reach for a half gallon of ice cream or a half pound burger. If you are lonely, go out to where people are and interact with them. Don't sit home with a bag of chips and a 2 liter soda.

I am not trying to make light of this. IN fact, I am trying to do exactly the opposite because this is such a problem with so many people. Food does not cure sadness and it doesn't make non-food issues better or worse. It is a coping mechanism and we must change that in order to control what we eat and what we weigh.

25. Stop Eating When You Start to Feel Full

This seems a little silly but for years I was doing something without even realizing it. I would eat and continue to eat until my plate was empty. I wasn't gorging myself or eating massive amounts of food, I was just eating a lot more than I really needed to without thinking about it. The result was packing on a few extra pounds each year.

I forget where I heard it but someone talked about being aware of how your body feels when you are eating and to stop eating when you felt full. Not when you feel bloated or stuffed, but instead just stop when you felt full. When you felt like you had eaten enough. It is a subtle feeling but you can definitely notice it if you just become aware of it.

I used to finish meals and feel really full sometimes to the [point of being really uncomfortable. I didn't "pig out" (although at times I might have) but after a few meals I would get that really uncomfortable feeling that I had just eaten too much.

But if you stop when you get that "I had enough" feeling, you will find that you are eating less, feeling better and losing some weight or at least gaining less. You are also doing your body a favor by not overloading your digestive system with huge amounts of food. If you are a diabetic you will also be lowering the demand for processing sugar which will help you keep your blood sugar levels more level.

26. Keep a Weight and Food Journal

Some people tend to think that this is a foolish or even stupid thing to do but keeping a weight journal can help you not only lose more weight but also help you identify activity or foods and how they affect your weight loss. Always remember that this is a long term process and not something that happens overnight.

Because it is a long term process, you will notice that certain things you do and certain things you eat will affect how much weight you lose or gain. Naturally, this information will be useful because we all want to do more of what makes us lose weight and less of what makes us gain weight. Cold, hard data and information can help us make the right decisions and create the right behaviors going forward.

Another powerful reason for keeping a journal is that sometimes when we look back at the end of the day those little "grabs" of food throughout the day can really add up. A few calories here and a few there can easily add up to several hundred calories a day. That can significantly impact our ability to reach our objectives.

I like to create the journal and write down everything I ate and whatever exercise I had during that day as well as what my weight was at the end of that day or whenever I weighed myself. This was handy because I then could easily look back and see what I did and ate on days where I lost weight and the same for days where I gained weight.

Moving forward, this gave me a reference or idea of what I had to do on any day that I wanted to lose weight. It also helped me established the level of exercise that I had to have to lose weight as well.

Trends are also important. If we see a trend where weight is slowly creeping up, this indicates a need to take a look at what we changed and make adjustments. This comes in handy after the holidays or after a vacation or during any time usually associated with weight gain.

While making the list will not alone help you gain or lose weight, it will give you the information you need to make better decisions and to better understand what needs to happen moving forward. It gives you accurate data relevant to YOU instead of generic data which might not pertain to your situation at all.

27. Don't Eat in Front of the TV

It seems that the world has gotten away from sitting down at the table for family meals. Instead, we set up a table in front of the television and eat our meals while watching TV. Not only does this keep us from communicating with each other on a regular basis, it also provides a way for us to consume more food without necessarily being aware of it.

Think about what happens when we eat in front of the TV. We are eating while watching the new or out favorite program that we taped or saved to the DVR. So we are concentrating not on what we're eating but also on what we're watching. The result is often eating faster but also eating more food than we usually would eat. That is because we are just not paying attention.

How many times have you sat at TV and snacked only to find that all of a sudden that bag of chips or cookies was all gone? You might have intended to only eat 3 or 4 cookies or handfuls of chips but instead you ate the whole bag. Not because you were a hog or wanted to but because you just were not paying attention. Plus, the food we usually eat at TV are not as nourishing or healthy as they would have been had we had a sit down meal with the family.

If you must eat in front of TV, or if you routinely eat alone and TV is your companion during meals, then fix your plate in the kitchen and do not bring entire bags or boxes of food to the couch with you. This will help you limit the amount of food you can eat without getting up to replenish your supply! This is like measuring your portions before you sit down!

28.   Try Leaner Cuts and Types of Meat

Sometimes we have food that aren't the best for us diet or health wise but we love them so much we are not willing to get rid of them. In these cases, we can try to get better versions of those foods to help us eat healthier and reduce calories.

For example, if you love beef or other red meat, try and eat leaner cuts of meat which will have less fat and therefore fewer calories. Not only is this a healthier alternative, you will be able to eat the meat you love without some of the calories.

Take chopped meat or hamburger, for example. You can get 75% beef which is 25% fat or you can get 85 or 90% beef which has lower amounts of fat. You can still have that burger you love but with the better cuts of meat you can ingest less fact and fewer calories. This will help your cholesterol and weight!

29.   Read the Damn Food Labels!

One of the best tools or weapons we have in our fight to lose weight are the same things many of us never bother to use in the first place! I am referring, of course, to the labels found on food containers and the calorie information placed on food service boards and restaurant menus. These alone can save us thousands of calories every week!

Recently I went to see a baseball game and went to order my usual popcorn because, well, popcorn is supposed to be a healthy snack, certain much better weight loss wise than cotton candy or a hot dog. But since my last visit they had placed calorie count on the menu board and I was blown away! The popcorn had 1,400 calories, the hot dog has 600 calories and the cotton candy, with all its sugar, was 250 calories!!!!!!

So my previously "healthy choice" was a diet killer! No, I realize cotton candy is the worse health-wise so I got the hot dog. I liked the hot dog and I liked the popcorn but knowing the calorie count enabled me to make the better choice and I went with the hot dog.

Read the labels on food products before you buy. Compare the calorie count and fat content so that you can choose the best products for your particular situation. Sometimes just changing to another brand can save you 100 calories. Just make sure to compare serving sizes as well so you get accurate information.

Labels provide us with extremely valuable information that we should always use when deciding which food products to eat. They are especially important when we are on a specific amount of calories per day. We then will know how many calories and what the serving size should be for everything we eat.

When it comes to eating out, hopefully the calories are listed on the menu. If they are, then take that into consideration. If your state does not require that, ask your representatives to get that into law. It really is a greater benefit to everyone trying to lose weight.

But always remember that when it comes to labels, they will not help you one damn bit if you don't use them. If the information is there but you don't read it, don't expect it to help you! So check the labels and choose and adjust what you are eating based on the information on the label.

30. Switch the White Bread for Whole Wheat

Whole wheat breads and flours use the entire grain whereas white bread and flour are processed and most of the nutrients, vitamins and minerals are removed during the processing.

This effects the amount of fiber in the food as well as making it far less nourishing for our bodies. Don't be fooled by seeing the term "enriched" in white four products such as bread. Whole wheat is still better for us and has more fiber which is needed for proper digestion.

31. Give Away Your "Larger" Clothes

We all have a pair of our "fat pants" in our closet. You know what I'm talking about. These are the pants we used to wear before we started losing weight. Hopefully now they are very loose on us and we have purchased new clothes in a smaller size. But when we keep those "fat pants" around, we are telling ourselves at some level that we might be back there in the future so we better hold on to them.

The problem with that attitude is that it makes it easier for us to backslide. If we find our newer clothes getting tight and we revert back to the larger sized clothes, we are removing an incentive or reminder that we are moving in the wrong direction. The result is that we continue moving in that wrong direction and gaining even more weight before we start once again turning things around.

If your older clothes are in great shape, consider donating them to the poor or to charities that help service and cloth the homeless. This way you put those older clothes to good use and people who need them can get use out of them. If those old clothes are not in great condition, consider just tossing them out or using them as rags the next time you are painting the living room or bedroom.

Do not use them as reminders of where you used to be or as a failsafe against getting back to your old weight in the future. Because if you give yourself that possibility, you are far more likely to take advantage of it.

32.　Stop Fast Food!

Obesity has increased every year over the last several decades and I cannot help but feel that it is because we make calorie rich food so more readily available now than it ever was before.

Unless you live in a rural area or small town you probably have several fast food places near you.

These places are convenient and while there is a spot for them in our culture, we have come to depend on them far too much for way too much of our diet. And this comes from me, someone who has eaten far more of their fair share of fast food in their lifetime!

There are two main problems with fast food when it comes to weight loss and dieting.

First of all, almost all fast food, even their so-called healthy choices" are much higher in calories than similar foods prepared at home. So you are eating higher calorie food which might be cheaper but also help you gain a ton of weight at the same time. These foods usually contain a ton of salt or sodium which is where they get there taste from as well. Since salt helps you retain water, it also helps you gain weight and also can raise your blood pressure at the same time!

Second, this type of food is just too convenient and provides us with an easy way of eating far too much. With all the "super sizes" out there we are encouraged to eat more than we should and along with that comes added calories and more weight. But the allure of getting food fast and not having to cook often comes out as being more important.

One thing that no one usually mentions but that I find very ironic, is that not only is most fast food not very nutritious, we don't even have to walk inside to get it.

We can sit our asses in the car and use the drive-thru! So we eat more calories and don't even have to walk the 30 steps to the counter to order it!

Be very careful even when it comes to so-called "healthy choices". Some of these are not as healthy as you might think. Be sure to ask for a nutrition pamphlet that lists calories and other data. Every fast food chain has them but sometimes you have to ask for it.

If you cannot eliminate fast food, do your best to severely limit it. Don't have it for lunch every day. If you want to splurge on a Friday to celebrate the end of the week, that's one thing. But downing a quarter pound burger, large fries and a super-sized 4 gallon cola is not going to help you lose weight any time soon.

33. Reduce Sodium

Since we were just talking about fast food, let's talk about reducing sodium. Although we all need a certain amount of sodium in our diets in order for our bodies to function normally, most of us get far too much sodium in our diets.

Fast food is one source for a HUGE amount of sodium. There is sodium in almost all the products and in restaurant sodium is used to give the dishes part of their flavor.

In some restaurants or bars they serve foods loaded with salt or sodium to make you thirstier so that you drink more and therefore purchase more drinks. That is marketing at its best!

Sodium is another line item on nutrition labels that we should pay attention to. Limiting the amount of sodium will help us retain less fluid and therefore lose weight faster. We should not eliminate ALL sodium from our diet because as we have already stated we need certain amounts of sodium for our bodies to function properly. But lowering sodium or salt intake should be on most of our lists.

Sodium causes us to retain more fluid which can lead to weight gain and higher blood pressure. I strongly urge everyone to discuss salt intake with their doctor as part of their yearly physical. It is a smart strategy for anyone looking to lose weight and eat healthier.

34.   Go for a Walk When You Get the Munchies

I get the munchies regularly and it can be very easy to blow a good day of dieting right out the window with one attack of the munchies. The next time a craving hits, instead of hitting the pantry for a bag of chips or a box of cookies, go for a walk instead. This will help you accomplish two things.

First, it will give you a chance to let the urges pass without hitting the snacks.

This will help you reduce the number of calories you eat and help you lose more weight in less time. Sometimes all we need to do is let the urge pass in order to avoid eating and that's is what our goal should be at first.

Second, by choosing exercise over eating, we are substituting a different behavior over eating. Exercising such as walking or running will burn calories as well. So even if we still have the munchies after a nice walk, we will probably eat less and will have burned off at least some of those calories during our exercise.

35.   Cut Back on Condiments

Here is a wake-up call for people who think no matter what they put on their food that condiments and spices have zero calories. I don't care what kind of food you put in your mouth, it is going to have calories in it. We might not be talking hundreds or thousands but we are still talking about calories and they all add up at the end of the week.

You cannot take a 500 calories burger and pile it high with lettuce, tomatoes, onions, sauces, ketchup, mayo, peppers and dressings and still have a 500 calorie burger! You could wind up with an 800 calorie burger or more!

One tablespoon of ketchup can add 20 calories, two tablespoons of some dressings can add 150 Calories! And a tablespoon is NOT a huge amount! Look at the amount of ketchup you could consume on French fries alone. You could easily add 200 calories to your meal!

Even a nice healthy plain green salad can become a high calorie meal if you add 1,000 calories worth of dressing and other items! I am not saying to eat everything plain and bland. But just be aware that everything you pour, drizzle, shake or dip on your food adds calories and those calories can quickly add up to extra pounds!

36. Get a Weight Loss Friend

If you really want to make weight loss easier, find a weight loss friend. That is someone who can lose weight along with you. Just having someone go through what you are going through with you can be motivating and supportive.

Not only that but one of the challenges people losing weight often have is interacting with people who either don't need to lose weight or just don't want to. So you go out to dinner and order you lightly dressed green salad while they scarf down wings, huge burgers and the hot fudge sundae for dessert! They don't do it because they want to be mean. They do it because they can and not gain weight.

But a weight loss buddy will also have that salad and will not tempt you or make your mouth water while looking at that sundae. When there is little or no temptation there is much less willpower involved.

Your weight loss buddy can also be someone that you can walk in the mornings with or join a gym together. They can also be the person you call when you have the munchies or really want to go through the drive through and get that milkshake and fries!

Never underestimate the value of having someone you can turn to for support and assistance. Just having someone there with you can greatly increase the odds of you being successful and sticking with your weight loss program. Plus, they can make it fun and more enjoyable at the same time. Since we tend to do things that are fun for longer periods of time, it just makes sense to make things as much fun and more enjoyable as possible.

When choosing a weight loss buddy, make sure you are compatible with one another. If you like hitting the gym 8 hours a day and run marathons, do not pick a buddy who likes a one mile leisurely walk around the neighborhood for their daily exercise. The same goes for food and diet as well. If you are a relaxed kind of person who wants to lose weight without a hardline approach, then pick a person with the same approach as your buddy.

Remember you goal should be to find someone to help you through the process not push you so hard you quit.

37.   Cut Back on TV

While I like TV as much as the next person, I do have to admit that sitting in front of a box watching sports is not nearly as good for losing weight as going out and PLAYING the same sport. But even if playing sports is not your goal, sitting around too much doing nothing but watching TV is not going to help you lose weight.

I do have a treadmill in an exercise room and I sometimes watch the news or programming while on the treadmill so that is OK. At least I am getting my cardio in at the same time I am watching TV. But to sit and watch TV all day long does no one any good.

I also realize that quitting TV cold turkey is not usually an option and quitting TV altogether is not reasonable either. So why not cut back one hour a day to start and substitute that one hour with a walk or workout? If you burn 200 calories in that one hour and you do that 7 days a week, then you will burn an extra 1,400 calories a week just by cutting TV down an hour a day.

If you must watch television, try and do so while moving around a bit. Even if it is something small you will burn calories. Lie on the floor and stretch or do leg lifts or anything that will burn a few calories. The more you do this sort of thing the less you will have to reduce calories or do other types of exercise and still lose weight.

38. Do 5 minutes Every Other Hour

While exercise is great in any form, we get the most benefit from exercise when we do it throughout the day. We should strive for at least 30-60 minutes of cardio at one time for cardio benefits but for the rest of our exercise, spreading it out throughout the day will help get our metabolism up and help it stay there.

Aim for at least 5-10 minutes of exercise every two hours. For most of us that will mean 8 or 9 periods of exercise during a normal day. This will enable us to keep our metabolism up and help us burn more calories. Plus, by keeping active throughout the entire day, we burn more calories and lose more fat.

It is also easier to burn the same amount of calories over several sessions than to try and do it all at once. This fits in very well with our philosophy of trying to come up with a plan we can live with for an extended period of time.

39. Use a Pedometer or Fitness Band

Some people think these fitness bands and other electronic devices are just fads and really don't do all that much to help us lose weight or get into better shape. I tend to disagree. IN fact, I feel that they can play a significant role in our weight loss.

One thing fitness bands and pedometers and other devices have in common is that they give us actual data on what we have done within a certain period of time. What this means is that we can accurately compare one day with another and also confirm that we actually did what we think we did instead of relying on guesswork or estimations.

For example, we might think we walked two miles during the day but if we had a pedometer we might find the actual distance to be 1 mile or 5 miles. Actual steps allow us to figure out exact distances and exercise. We can use pedometers to help make sure that we walk at least a certain amount every day using the pedometer as a reference.

Fitness bands are more complex devices that provide not only numbers of steps but also some measurement of physical exertion. The level of activity is important because you will burn more energy and calories running for 3,000 steps than you would walking 3,000 steps. So the level of activity is important as well as the length or duration of the activity. Fitness bands will allow you to more accurately track the total amount and intensity of exercise.

One thing that I find useful with pedometers or fitness bands is that you can see later in the day exactly where you stand as far as exercise that day. If you are close to goal that's great. But if you are really behind your daily goal you can go for an after dinner walk or go to the gym to catch up on what you couldn't or didn't do during the day.

Some fitness bands will also track how many hours you were active for at least 5 minutes during that hour. That helps us spread our activity more evenly throughout the day to keep our metabolism as high as it can be.

Fitness bands also let you track performance over days, weeks and months. If you are into this and like to see your improvement or lack of, this might be of interest to you. Otherwise, just use your pedometer or fitness band to make sure you hit your daily targets.

Which device should you get? It depends on what you want to do with it. Pedometers are cheaper and will allow you to tack and set step goals for every day. For many of us that will be enough. If you want to measure or track intensity or other things, then perhaps a fitness band is the way to go.

But regardless of which device you get, it will only be as useful as you allow it to be. If you buy a pedometer but never look at it, it will be a waste.

The same with a fitness band. But if you establish goals and use either device to help you achieve them, they can be a great help in getting you to where you want to go.

40.   Change from Whole Milk to 1 or 2%

Here's an easy one. If you drink milk, switch to one of the lower fat versions. If you like whole milk, try 2% milk. If you are using 2% consider going to 1% milk. Depending on which version you are using now, switching to 1 or 2% can save you 20% in calories!

You can try switching the type of milk you use in cooking but should be aware that fat content does play a certain part in some recipes so changing the milk might have an effect on the taste of the final product.

41.   Shop on a Full Stomach!

You might laugh at this one but it's really true. If you go shopping when you are hungry, you will tend to buy more junk food and snacky and rich foods. The ice cream bars will look better, the chips taste better and all sorts of baked goods and other things somehow will wind up in your cart.

You are far better off going shopping right after you eat when you are the least hungry.

It might be easier or more convenient stopping on the way home from work before dinner but that could result in a whole pantry full of comfort foods.

I have tried this personally and I was shocked at the difference. Once I went shopping when I was not feeling well and I hardly bought a thing! But you don't have to be sick to shop better. You just need to be full!

42.   When Shopping, Perimeter Shop!

Some people might not be aware of this but the healthier foods are generally around the perimeter of the store so if you do most of your shopping around the perimeter you should do better. The exception to this are stores that place sale items on the end caps of the aisles. In those stores you can find all kinds of stuff on or around the perimeter of the store.

43.   Cook More, Take-In Less!

OK< don't shoot the messenger here but when you cook meals at home you generally consume fewer calories. That is because you have direct control over what you make and how you make it.

You can cook low fat versions of your favorite foods. You can use no-salt or low-salt recipes to limit the amount of salt that is in the foods you eat.

You can also create healthier meals using healthier things to go along with them.

You can also limit portion size by just cooking enough for you or the two of you. This way you can have a normal sized burger and enjoy it without having to order the 12 ounce gigunda burger with its 2,000 calories! Even if you wanted fries you can bake a small amount of them in the oven and save on the fat and calories.

Eating fewer calories does not always mean suffering and not eating the foods you love. Sometimes it just means preparing those foods yourself so you can take control of ingredients and portion size.

As an added bonus it is usually much cheaper to eat home as well. You could even use some of that money you saved towards purchasing some new clothes to fit the skinnier you!

44.   Don't Keep Food Out Where You Can See It!

Our brains are very visual organs. Our eyes see things and rely that information and when it comes to food, what our eyes see our brain wants. So if you have a bowl of candy sitting on the table next to you, it is far more likely that you will have a few pieces (or more!) while you are sitting there than if it wasn't there to remind you.

The old saying "out of sight, out of mind" is very true. We will tend to want what we see and sometimes forget about what we don't see. So if you have to have some food on display or near you make it a bowl of fruit and not a bowl of candy. Every little bit helps when it comes to control impulse eating and binges!

45. Make Smaller Goals

If you have a weight loss goal, then good for you! It is much easier to achieve a goal if you identify what that goal is in the first place. But sometimes a large goal can be so intimidating that we sometimes give up before we really get started. Because of this we need to rethink the way we set our goals.

If you want to lose 5 pounds, then set your goal at 5 pounds. It is not that intimidating. But if you need to lose 50 pounds, or even 100 pounds, goals that large can be thought or us extremely difficult if not impossible to achieve. In these cases, we need to break up our larger goals into smaller and more attainable ones. We need to do this for several reasons.

First, as we already said, very large goals can be intimidating. We want to avoid that and make our goals appear closer and easier to achieve than they might actually be. It's a mind game at some times and it's a mind game we need to win in order to be successful.

Second, smaller goals are more motivating. When you have a 5 pound goal and lose one pound you are 20% there! But if you need to lose 100 pounds and you lose one pound, you are only 1% there. That is a huge difference! When the end of the tunnel appears closer we become more motivated.

So let's break up that 100 pound goal into 10 ten pound goals or maybe even 20 five pound goals. This will enable us to get more excited and more motivated as we achieve each of those 5 or 10 milestones. While you are not losing more weight or losing it any faster, it appears that you are making more or better progress and that's a good thing.

Anyone experienced in any form of goal setting will tell you that it is important that any goal be considered achievable. By making our goals appear easier and more achievable we increase the likelihood of turning those goals into reality!

46.   Have More Sex!

Do you want a fun way to lose weight? Try having more sex! Sexual activity not only is fun and enjoyable, it also burns calories! Depending on the type of activity, you might burn a few hundred calories while having a great time doing it!

Another benefit is that the time you spend having sex reduces the time you have to just sit around and do nothing.

Even better, sex counts as cardio activity and exercise as well! So you get to have fun, get another exercise session, burn calories and improve your relationship all at the same time!

We really don't have to go into more detail on this one. It is pretty self-explanatory! But a word of caution. If you use whipped cream during sex remember that it has calories!

47. Reward Yourself Along the Way!

Losing weight is not that different from anything else in life that we accomplish. Since we often celebrate accomplishments in life, celebrating your weight loss should be celebrated as well!

Now we don't mean eating a 5 scoop ice cream sundae or wolfing down a one pound burger, but there is nothing wrong with going out and buying a new outfit or a new tool or something you like.

In fact, set a reward for yourself as an added incentive for achieving a certain goal. Tell yourself you will go out and buy a new outfit once you have lost 20 pounds. Or that you will buy yourself that new cordless drill you want when you hit your goal!

If you know someone who is trying to lose weight, why not offer them an incentive as well? Don't push them or hound them but tell them you will take them to a movie or a night out once they have hit their goal. Whatever you can do to provide motivation or an incentive then go ahead and try it!

48.   Use Smaller Plates

This is another one of those "silly" tips that really work. Using smaller plate helps us accomplish two things.

First, smaller plates hold less food so that means you won't be able to hold as many calories on one plate. So this is a perfect way to downsize portions and use portion control to limit the calories you eat.

Second, smaller plates get full faster and a full plate looks like more food than a half full plate. Even if you place the exact same amount of food on two plates, the food on the smaller plate will appear to be more food. Since so much of how we interpret things is based on what our eyes see, the smaller plate will make us think we are eating a larger amount of food!

49.   Learn to Deal with Stress

Stress is not a friend of the person trying to lose weight.

Stress causes us to seek food as a comfort and is one of the most common sources of binging and cheating on your diet. The key to beating stress and sticking to your diet is replacing the way you address the stress in your life.

As we said already earlier in this book, substituting another behavior for eating when we are under stress will help us stay faithful to our diet. Instead of binging, take a walk or go to the gym. Instead of keeping things inside us, let them out and take out your frustrations at the gym or by taking a quick run.

The key to getting control over stress is eliminating most root causes of stress in your life. That means making life easier and less stressful by having people around you that help make your life better instead of causing you stress. It means identifying the things that bring stress and either changing them or getting rid of them.

Often times this is as simple as letting go of the little things in life that cause you stress but aren't really worth it. In other words, don't sweat the small stuff so much and instead concentrate on what really is important to you in life. You will find yourself not only losing weight easier but enjoying life a whole lot more in the process!

50.   Stay Away from Enablers

As you go through your life you will see that there will be people who help us achieve our goals and those who will do their best to keep us from the things in life that we want. In other words, there will be people who will help us succeed or enable us to fail. The good news is that we are almost always able to choose who we will associate with.

Most of our real friends will support us as we try to lose weight. But other people, who might have their own agenda and reasons for seeing you fail, will try to lead us astray from our goals. It really doesn't make much difference why they want us to fail, all that matters is that we recognize what they are trying to do.

If you find in your case that there are people who are trying to tempt you or lead you away from your goals, stop associating with those people. Instead, seek out people who want to help you make your life better even though it might not be in their best interests to do so. Those are your real friends.

You might find that you're over weight friends do not wish to see you lose weight because that will make them less attractive or they might feel that once you lose the weight that you will abandon them. Though you might understand their reasons, you should not allow them to keep you from achieving you goals.

Talk to those people and make them understand that losing weight is important to you and that it will not affect your friendship with them. Give them a chance to come around to your point of view. If they do come around, that's great. If they still stand between you and your goals, it might be time to look for new friends or at least limit your time around them

Only you can determine what action would be in your best interests. Once you decide, then do not hesitate to do what is in your best interest. You are your own best advocate and you need to take control over your life and your future.

51.   Use the Tape NOT Just the Scale!

I know we talked about the reasons and need for weighing yourself regularly as a means of identifying good and bad behaviors and habit and what their effect was on our weight loss. But there are other ways to measure weight loss that need to be done in addition to stepping on the scale every day.

As we exercise and lose weight, some fat will be replaced by muscle. While that is good, fat weighs less than muscle so as muscle replaces fat you might not lose weight and you might even gain a bit! But this can be a good thing!

Use a tape measure to keep track of your waist measurement and other measurements as well. Added muscle in the legs and chest can alter your weight and cause you to think that you are not making much progress even though you might be making great progress!

Let me ask you, if you went on a diet and didn't weigh yourself for 6 months but you went from a 40 inch waist down to a 34 inch waist, would you consider that making progress? Of course you would. If you are looking better and feeling better and your body is more defined and well-toned, that is more important than the scale.

So use the scale along with the measuring tape to get a better and more accurate idea of how well you are doing and how much progress you are making. It is not just the pounds that matter. It is how you look and feel about yourself that makes all the difference!

52.   Drink Green Tea

Green tea is said to boost metabolism and be a great weight loss aid. If you enjoy drinking tea, then switch to green tea which is supposed to be healthier and better for you than regular tea.

As far as weight loss is concerned, there are green tea extract supplements out there that are supposed to increase metabolism and allow you to lose more weight faster. Whether they will work for you or not remains to be seen. But always remember that these pills and drinks are no substitute for a medically sound diet designed for weight loss.

53. Don't Super Mega-Size Your Drinks!

For many people, sugary drinks are the worst part of their caloric intake. They go to the local convenience store and buy the 4 gallon soft drink and sip it all day or at least until lunch when they go out and get another one for the afternoon.

But consider that a 32 ounce drink, commonly called a large in some fast food places, can have 400-500 calories in it! That means it is easy to consume 1,000 calories a day in soft drinks alone! There is no way anyone consuming that much sugar and calories in just soft drinks is going to lose weight and still have a healthy diet!

Over the years soft drink sizes have gradually been getting larger. Small drinks today used to be called medium a few years back. It has gotten so bad that the large cups are so large that it is difficult to hold them with one hand!

It is really crazy because if someone told you they had 3 or 4 cans of soda with a meal, you would think they are crazy. But that is exactly what those 32 ounce or larger drinks are! 3 cans of soda contain 36 ounces!

Even consuming diet soda in such large quantities is not smart because of all the artificial sweeteners used in them.

Even though they have very few calories it is not good to put so much artificial stuff in your body every day. If you must have soda, make it a diet soda and even then in moderation.

The best beverage to drink is plain old water. It will hydrate you properly and help your body flush out toxins and waste products properly making you feel better and lighter. Most people are not aware of it but a lot of soft drinks contain a lot of salt. They contain salt because it helps make you thirsty and what do you do when you are thirsty? You buy a larger drink. It's a vicious cycle everyone needs to break!

54.   Have a Shopping List Handy!

If you have to go shopping, create a list before you go and then stick to that list. Go from item to item and then get out of the store. Do not walk up and down the aisles looking for what looks good! Because if you do that your cart will be full of stuff you shouldn't be eating and stuff you will regret eating immediately after finishing it!

Anything that helps us get what we need and get out fast without buying fattening or high calorie comfort food is the way to go. Remember, if it isn't available to us at home we can't eat it unless we go out and buy it. We cannot eat what we do not have!

55.   Handle Set-backs Better!

When we are trying to lose weight we need to handle set-backs properly. We all know about set-backs because EVERYONE experiences them at some time during the weight loss process. When they happen how we deal with them will often mean the difference between success and failure.

Set-backs are days, or even weeks, when we do not lose weight but in fact gain some. We all have times when this happens. A big party or wedding reception, a vacation at an all-inclusive resort or the entire holiday season where we are surrounded by big meals, snacks and treats. Everyone has these events in their lives so it is not a case of whether we will have set-backs but when they are going to occur.

Some people get discouraged by a set-back and think all is lost and just give up. They figure things are too hard and they just can't do it anyone. They fear all is lost and just become too frustrated to continue. Then they abandon what had worked up until then and go back to their old ways and the weight they lost soon returns with a vengeance.

The best way to handle a set-back is just accept it and move on. If you had followed a previous tip and created a food and exercise journal, you will be able to easily see why you had the set-back.

You might know anyway but actually seeing it written down drives the real reason home. As we said before, hard data is always better than a perception.

Whether you had a journal or not, just sit back and think things through. Understand why the set-back occurred and remember what had worked for you up until that point. Then commit yourself to returning to that behavior and diet. Chances are if you are able to do that you will be successful in continuing to lose weight until you reach your goal.

56.   Take a Picture or Two

We talked a while back about the need to get motivated and stay motivated. Weight loss is rarely an easy process nor is it a quick one either. But if we are able to remain motivated throughout the process we stand a much better chance of losing the weight we want to lose.

One way to get motivated is to take a picture of you that really highlights what you really look like under those clothes. Take a picture in a bathing suit or other clothes that do not hide your body. If you want to take a naked picture, then go ahead but a bathing suit will do just fine and those pictures you can share with others afterwards if you want!

As you go through the weight loss process, take the same picture in the same clothes or bathing suit at various stages of weight loss.

Use the same pose or close to it and take the picture from the same distance and angle. What you want to be able to see is the difference in how you look as the weight comes off.

We all have seen before and after pictures of people who have undergone some kind of transformation and those people have those pictures for the same reason as we are suggesting them now. They used them to feel good about themselves and so that they could see the results of their efforts. Sometimes things might not show up on a scale or even a tape measure but you can see them easily in a picture.

Whatever gets and keeps you motivated is good for you!

57. Forget Miracle Cures and Fads

I saved this one for one of the last ones because I didn't want to burst your bubble and get you discouraged. But at this point you have read over 50 ways that you can use to help you lose the weight you want or need to lose. So at this point you should realize that you can do this and that it can be easier than you originally thought. So now is the perfect time to talk about something that doesn't work.

If you look at any health magazine or mainstream publication or television talk shows you will see article after article about fad diets and amazing diet pills.

They promise rapid weight loss without dieting or without exercise. They seem too good to be true and most of the time, they are. I say "most of the time" so I don't get my ass sued by someone who does have something that actually does work!

I have seen plastic suits that you sleep in that make you sweat so you appear to lose weight but it is just water weight that you put back on as soon as you start drinking water again. I had seen water diets, low carb diets, low fat diets, special exercise equipment and a host of other things designed to make your wallet lighter first with only a possibility of making you lighter in the process.

As you look at any of these diets and exercise gizmos, remember one universal truth when it comes to weight loss. You can only lose weight when your body uses more calories per day than it takes in. If you eat less calories than your body uses in a day, you will lose weight. If you consume more calories than your body burned in a day, you will gain weight. That is true for all of us.

So anything that makes us burn more calories or eat less calories will enable us to lose weight. As far as those exercise gizmos are concerned, they might work because they get you to move and movement burns calories. I don't care which piece of equipment you use, if you use that instead of sitting on the couch watching television you will burn more calories!

If you look close at the disclaimer on the commercial or the box the gizmo came in, it will say that you will lose weight using this equipment AND a responsible reduced calorie diet,

DUH! If you reduce the calories you eat enough you will lose weight!

The problem with fads and gizmos is that they might work for the short-term but they can produce risks to your health and your ability to keep the weight off. Remember that we are losing weight to be healthier but if the methods we use to lose that weight are unhealthy by themselves we are defeating the purpose of losing the weight in the first place. In some cases we can do more harm than good!

As far as pills and supplements are concerned, some of them might work for you. If they raise your metabolism and help you burn more calories, then they could help you lose weight. But those pills that are supposed to make you lose 30 pounds in a month without diet or exercise I would be very skeptical about.

Let me leave you with one thought regarding weight loss supplements and magic pills. If there was a pill or supplement that really helped you lose massive amounts of weight without diet or exercise, do you think they would sell it for $9.95 in the corner supermarket or vitamin store?

No, if it really worked like magic then they would be getting top dollar for it because a pill like that could actually change your life. Again, stuff might work but you really need to be careful when it comes to putting substances into your body.

But let's move on to more about this.

58.   Always Go Healthy

Though a lot of people try to lose weight to improve the way they look or to fit into smaller clothes, an important component to weight loss is an improvement in our health. Losing weight allows us to place less strain on our bones and muscles while lower weight can sometimes reduce our blood pressure as well. Since high blood pressure often has no symptoms and can cause serious health issues, anything we can do to lower it will be beneficial. So no matter what the reason you have for losing your weight, let's agree there are also medical and health benefits as well.

But sometimes the way we go about losing weight can cause even worse health issues for us. Starvation diets, dangerous or harmful pills or supplements and too much exercise can often hinder our efforts to continue our effort and might even cause significant health issues.

No don't think for even a minute that this gives you a reason to stop trying to lose weight!

We are not talking about stopping our efforts! We are talking about doing things I a healthy and responsible manner. The first step in any weight loss program is to stop by and see your doctor.

Your doctor should be the one to guide you on how to best go about losing weight. Chances are he will tell you to reduce the number of calories you are eating each day and to add some exercise. But he will also give you some guidelines as to what is medically safe for you. This will depend on your age, overall physical condition and any health problems or issues that you might have.

The last thing we want to do is hurt ourselves by doing too much too soon. While aches and pains are normal, exercising to the point of tearing a muscle or causing severe pain will not help us. It will just force us to stop until we heal. Instead we want to create a responsible diet and exercise program that has the approval and blessing of our doctor. He will likely want to see you throughout your program to check your progress and monitor your health.

When you go to your doctor to talk about your weight loss program, please listen to what he says and follow it to the letter. Don' think you can do more because more is better. A responsible diet is one thing but a starvation diet is not better, it is much worse.

You and your doctor should come up with a program that will help you accomplish your goals while at the same time be something you can stick with for an extended period of time. Any program that requires too much effort or extreme sacrifice is just not going to be sustainable. Aim for something you can stick with and concentrate on that.

59.　Have a Weigh-In

We have all heard of these weight loss programs where you go to meetings where you get weighed in every week to check your progress. Some people wonder why the meeting are necessary and most of us think it is because of the speakers and lecturers who teach us how to lose weight the right way. While part of that is true, there is a bigger reason why the meeting format seems to work for so many. The weigh-in.

People do not like to show others that they failed to live up to their commitments. Everyone likes to succeed and no one likes to admit defeat in front of others. Sometimes just the fear of standing up in front of people and revealing that you gained a pound over the last week is enough to stop people from over eating or binging. They just do not want to stand up in front of a bunch of people and show a weight gain.

This is all about motivation. In this case it is the fear of admitting failure that motivates people to keep up their diet and exercise program for another week.

But most of us don't need a meeting setting to get the same benefits. If you are exercising with others why not stage your own weekly weigh-in? This way you will all be motivated to stick to the program and you can eliminate the weekly meeting fees.

If you are married or living with someone, have a weekly weigh-in with your spouse or partner. This can help you stay motivated as well. Just make sure you choose people who will not judge you or make fun of you when you do have a set-back. The focus must always remain on the positive while dealing with whatever negatives might come about. All motivation must be positive in nature to continue helping us.

60.   Attitude Adjustment

Successful long-term weight loss is more than just a diet and exercise program. It also requires an attitude adjustment. If you don't change the way you look at eating and exercise you might lose the weight but it will come back. You cannot expect to lose 100 pound, then return to your old ways, and expect that weight to stay off. It just doesn't work that way!

In order to sustain weight loss and then keep the weight off, we j=must change the way we live. We must change our lifestyle and the way we use food in our lives. We need to change our response to stress and negative situations.

We must avoid comfort eating and binge eating and substitute other behaviors.

In other words, we must change the way we think about life, food and weight. If we can manage to do that we will find ourselves eating better, eating healthier and losing the weight we wanted to lose. Then we will be able to sustain that weight loss and not gain any of it back over the next few years. When can manage to accomplish this, our goals will stay achieved.

61.   Act Your Age!

Let's have a bit of a reality check right now. If you are in your 20's and looking to lose weight, God bless you. As long as your doctor agrees, the sky is probably the limit as far as what you can do is concerned. Just be reasonable and responsible.

But if you are in your 50's or older, we must stop back and remind ourselves that we are no longer in our 20's. We simply cannot do what we used to do 20 or 30 years ago and we should not expect our bodies to do those things. If we are older than our 50's this becomes more and more of a reality.

As we age our bodies require more and more time to rebound or recover from the things we do. Not only that but our muscles become weaker and our bones a little bit more brittle. We might be able to get through the day just fine but we can no longer run as fast or for as long as we used to. This doesn't mean we are out of shape or anything sometimes, it just means we are older and our bodies have aged a bit.

The older we are the more careful we need to be. We are not invincible as we used to think we are. We can still do a lot, though it we are responsible about it. Seeing our doctor is even more important as we get older. Taking into consideration our overall physical health and condition becomes more important as well.

We also might have to adjust the way we exercise as well. While we used to run to get into shape we might have to switch to walking now. The main point is to not stop exercising as we get older but instead switch to a more appropriate form of exercise.

For example, if we used to lift free weights, as we get older we might want to switch to weights on machines in the gym so we do not have to worry about dropping weights should they become too heavy. Maybe it means dialing back the speed on the treadmill to a slightly slower speed and walk a bit longer instead. We even might decide to get a personal trainer to help us make the transition to exercising in a different manner as we get older.

Just because we get older doesn't mean we should stop exercising. Exercise helps us stay and feel young when we do it the right and responsible way. So don't stop exercising, just do what you are capable of as often as you can. If you can do that, you will do just fine.

59.   Don't go Back!

One of the problems a lot of people have after they lose the weight is keeping that weight off for long period of time. For many people losing weight is often accompanied by putting that weight back on often with even more weight. This usually happens for one important reason.

We lost the weight but did not change our attitude towards eating and weight loss. In other ways, we went back to our old ways. The problem with this is when we lose weight and then gain it back this can cause severe health issues sometimes even greater than if we hadn't lost the weight in the first place!

This kind of weight loss and gain is usually referred to as "yo-yo" dieting where our weight goes up and down like a yo-yo. We lose 10 pound, put back on 15 pound, lose that 15 pounds and gain back 20 and so on. This is not only frustrating for us, it can cause health issues as well.

The best way to avoid yo-yo dieting is to be aware of your current weight and maintain that weight. If you see a pound or two creep back on, make changes right then and there to stop that trend. Don't let one pound become 5 or 10. Stop weight gain quickly. This will make maintaining the weight easier and less stressful.

The best way to transition from weight loss to maintaining weight is to gradually change from losing weight mode to a maintenance mode where you allow yourself to eat SLIGHTLY more but not enough to allow weight gain.

For example. If you were on a 1,500 calorie diet to lose weight you might change to a 1,800 calorie diet to keep the weight off.

You cannot be on a 1,500 calorie diet to lose weight, achieve your goal and then start eating 3,500 calories a day and expect to keep that weight off. Always remember that what didn't work before is not going to work now either. You cannot go back to your old ways and expect different results!

Weight yourself often and keep a journal of your weight so you can spot trends and problems faster and easier. When you see something moving in the wrong direction make adjustments quickly to minimize the damage. Even more important, discover any damaging behavior or attitudes and change those attitudes so they will no longer cause weight gain and other problems.

62.   Don't Be Afraid to Ask for Help!

A lot of people are embarrassed to admit that they need help. They feel that admitting they need help is a sign of weakness. But the fact is, admitting you need help and asking for it is a measure of strength not weakness. But despite this, many people will not seek the help that they need and because of that will never reach their goals.

Help is available for weight loss in many forms. That is because people gain weight for many different reasons. There could be medical or psychological reasons or people might just like to eat more than they should. There could be environmental reasons as well. Whatever your reasons might be, you need to uncover them, understand them and deal with them.

Reaching out to your doctor is a great place to start. He or she can help you from the medical and health aspects of losing weight. They can provide you with responsible diets and even recommend other professionals that can help you out with other aspects such as exercise and attitudes. Whether you feel you need help or not, your doctor should always be the first place to start before starting any weight loss plan.

If there are emotional or psychological issues that are the cause or might be contributing to your weight problems, consulting a therapist might be important for you as well. There is no shame in doing this nor should you be embarrassed. Getting to the root cause of any problems is critical to being able to resolve the problem quickly and effectively. If you have problems with stress or emotional eating, this might be the perfect place to start.

For others joining a weight loss program with scheduled meetings might be a great place to get the support you need. Sometimes just hearing other people with the same problems talk might make you feel that you are not alone or weak because there are others with the same problems and issue that you have.

Hearing and learning how they managed to overcome certain things might give you the ideas or inspiration that you need to accomplish the same things in your life. If you feel that you might benefit from this sort of help, join one of the local programs available in your area.

Other people might have all the good intentions in the world but lack the knowledge to create a good and effective program. As we said your doctor would be a great place to start. But if you don't know how to cook a great meal, maybe consulting a nutritionist would be a great place to start. They can get you started in eating healthy and responsibly.

If exercising is something you need help with, why not take a class or arrange a few sessions with a personal trainer to learn the right way to exercise and to have a program designed for you specifically. You don't have to keep on seeing the trainer if you don't want to. Just do a few sessions to learn the correct form and how to do the various exercises and then continue on your own. Most gyms have trainers on staff and you can hire them on a single session basis or sign up for a complete program. They choice is yours.

Last but not least, for those who need information and do not want to get others involved for whatever reason, books like these are great ways to get the information you need both to get you started and to learn things you never even thought of.

Different books will give you different views on the same topics and you can read a few books and use what applies to your own situation so that you can develop the best plan for you.

Regardless of where you get the help you need, the important thing is to go get that help. Once you have the help in place, listen to what they are telling you and be open minded. The most important step is accomplishing anything or creating any type of change is to be honest with yourself. Don't try and convince yourself that you are different than you really are. You are only fooling yourself.

63.   It's Up to You Now!

At this point we have covered just about everything you will need to get started losing the weight you want to use. We have talked about why you should lose the weight, given you over 50 ways to lose that weight and have talked about support, motivation and a variety of other things all geared to you and your weight loss. In other words, we have given you the information and tools you need to accomplish your weight loss goals.

But now it is up to you. You know how to do what you need to do and you know how to get started. You know how to evaluate what you are doing and how effective or ineffective it is going for you. You are in the driver's seat and you are in control. That's the good news.

If there is any bad news in the above statement is that because you are in the driver's seat and the one that is in control, you are also the one responsible for the outcome. We can show you how to eat properly and lose weight. But only you control whether or not that hot fudge sundae goes from a thought in your head to a reality in your stomach.

We say this not to make you feel bad or to pressure you but instead to give you the last, and potentially most important aspect of weight loss and weight control. If you want to succeed in weight loss or anything in life you need to take responsibility for your actions. That means owning what you do, how you think, and how you react.

It is important to take responsibility for things because when we do that we tend to think about things differently. If all we do is make excuses then we fail to take things seriously and the role we play in those things.

If we constantly blame co-workers for our weight gain because someone brings donuts into the office every day then we will never realize that it is up to use whether we eat those donuts or not. So we keep eating them and we keep gaining weight or fail to lose any weight.

But if we take responsibility and really understand that it is our fault because no one forces us to eat those donuts that is when we make a real changes that enable us to achieve real results!

Because when we change things, things change. That is a simple statement with very real meaning.

Taking responsibility for things places us in the frame of mind to look at things from a different standpoint. We no longer feel sorry for ourselves but instead look for things we can do to make the outcome. We realize that just because those donuts are sitting there does not mean we have to look at them and eat them. Instead we might simply change the location of them so we don't see them.

It is also important to understand that we cannot always control the actions of others. We might ask people not to bring in the donuts but unless we own the business we cannot force them to obey your wishes. People will always find ways to do the things they want to do. So we have to approach things differently.

We need to understand that the only person that we have control over is ourselves. We have the ability to control what we do and how we react. We have control over what goes into our mouths and when we go to the gym or for a walk. We cannot force others to do what we want but we can force ourselves to do what we know needs to be done.

So from this minute on, take responsibility for everything you think and do. Take responsibility for what you eat, how and when you exercise and for any weight you lose or gain. Because once you do that, you open up a whole new world of options and alternatives each of which can help you get closer and closer to your goals.

This is not about anyone else or what anyone else thinks about you. It is about what you think of yourself and what you want out of life. If you want something for yourself, you have to go out and grab it. Things happen to people who go after what they want in life.

So if you want to lose weight then you need to go out and do it. Ask for help and involve others if that's what it takes but always believe and understand that the final responsibility of what you do always lies within you.

Once you reach that point, everything become much easier and you usually get much better results as well!

For more information on weight loss and other topics, please go to our website at:

http://www.26ways.com

While you are there, please take a moment to sign up for our mailing list.

It's free and there is no obligation to purchase anything. Members get free books, information and more free resources.

It's free, it's confidential and we will never share, rent or sell your information to anyone for any reason.